Black Garlic

Heinz   Guenther Saenger

Book Description

Some foods have all the good fortune! Not only does the flavor of black garlic take your taste buds on an unforgettable journey, but it also offers a wide range of positive effects on your body.

The mysterious history and benefits of "black garlic" have a great deal of ambiguities around them, and Heinz Guenther Saenger wants to clear all of that out in his book. Black garlic, which is highly prized in modern-day Japan, Thailand, and Korea, is a relative newcomer to the mainstream market in the United States (since about 2008). It is becoming more well-known these days for both the unique flavor it imparts and the beneficial effects it has on one's health.

The fact that black garlic contains almost twice as many antioxidants and nutrients as raw garlic means that it can treat circulation issues, heart disease, inflammation, age-damaged skin, high cholesterol level, diabetes, impaired immune system, cancer, liver damage, Alzheimer's disease, and other chronic disorders.

The benefits of this black gold shouldn't be hidden any longer, agree? Let's explore this nutrient-dense food!

Der Autor:

Born on 27.08.1956 in Hirzenhain, since 01.06.2021
Retired. Married in second marriage with Nittaya
Prommun.

Two daughters from first marriage

Black Garlic

Introduce Yourself with Black Garlic's
Miraculous Qualities

from

Heinz   Guenther Saenger

1. Impressum

1. Edition, 2022

© 2022 All rights reserved.

No. 4/2 Moo 7, A. Muaeng Ban Khok 67000

Phetchabun / Thailand

hgs56@ymail.com

2. © Copyright 2022 by Heinz Guenther Saenger - All rights reserved.

The goal of this book is to offer accurate and reliable information about the subject at hand. The publisher is not obligated to provide accounting, legally authorized, or otherwise qualifying services. If legal or technical advice is required, a knowledgeable expert should be contacted.

3. Table of Contents

BLACK GARLIC

4. Introduction

There are many miracles in the world to be celebrated
and, for me, garlic is the most deserving.

–Leo Buscaglia

The usage of black garlic dates back hundreds of years.
It was first marketed as a health product, and many
people still consider it to be a dietary supplement for
improved health. Every year, people in the United
States eat more than 250 million pounds of garlic. In
addition, it is very well-liked in the nations of the
Middle East and the Mediterranean, in addition to
China and India. In Thailand, locals have a strong belief
that using black garlic would make them live longer.
Since 2008, it has been slowly making its way into the
mainstream in the United States. Because of its complex
taste that combines sweet and savory flavors, it is
highly sought after by renowned chefs[1].

The culture of Korea, which is most well-known for its
kimchi, has refined the technique of fermenting by
slowly elevating the tastes of common foods to a whole
new level. It should come as no surprise that Korea was
the country where black garlic first appeared. After
being aged for at least a month, it has a caramelized
sweetness, savory richness, and a tongue feel that is
comparable to that of eating a date. It is both sweet and
mellow, making it difficult to realize that you are really
consuming garlic. These fermented cloves have a
smooth texture and they are simple to eat on their own

and do not leave a strong aftertaste in the mouth. Over the last few years in the whole world, we've seen that it's been showing up more and more often, and now it's back at the top of many seasonal, must-have ingredient lists at the very finest restaurants and now even at pizza places.

The fermentation process of black garlic is easy and natural, and it does not involve the use of any preservatives. The end product is even more nutritious than conventional garlic that has not been fermented. It's been said that black garlic has twice as many antioxidants and vitamin C as regular garlic, so there's really no reason not to like it.

Garlic, in all of its forms, is an effective natural medication. While black garlic may have a little more of an allure as a flavor enhancer in food, don't forget that it can be eaten raw. It is a powerful antibiotic as well as an antiviral agent, and it may be used to assist in the treatment of a wide variety of illnesses. In addition to this, it includes compounds that are helpful to fight against cancer. The fact that black garlic has so many positive effects on one's health—including lowering cholesterol levels, improving immunological function, reducing the onset of chronic illnesses, and a host of other advantages—has contributed to its meteoric rise in popularity. In addition to this, it is a wonderful source of antioxidants and vitamins, both of which are essential for maintaining the health of the body[2]. Let's explore more about this super-food!

5. Chapter 1.

What Is Black Garlic

Black garlic is aged fresh garlic that has a smooth, soft texture and a rich, sweet taste. It may be used to enhance the flavor of a wide variety of savory dishes (and even some sweet ones!). Black garlic also has a darker color than regular fresh garlic. Cloves of black garlic may be minced, crushed, or pureed with relative ease, making them an excellent addition to sauces, stews, pasta, and sautéed vegetables.

Nutrition profile

The following nutrients can be found in 15 grams of peeled black garlic[3]:

- Calories: 40

- Protein: 2 grams

- Fat: 0 grams

- Carbohydrates: 8 grams

- Fiber: 3 grams

- Sugar: 4 grams

Additionally, black garlic has detectable levels of the following:

- Vitamin C

- B Vitamins (B1, B2, B3, B6)

- Folate

- Calcium

- Manganese

- Magnesium

- Phosphorous

- Zinc

- Iron

Black garlic has a lower concentration of the chemical known as allicin, which is responsible for many of the positive health effects that are associated with ordinary garlic. However, it has a high concentration of phytonutrients, amino acids, and antioxidants. The concentrations, on the other hand, shift as a result of the aging process.

The antioxidant content of black garlic is higher than that of ordinary garlic. In addition to that, it has a greater quantity of a substance known as S-Allylcysteine (SAC). Allicin is more easily absorbed by the body thanks to SAC. Because it contains more allicin than regular garlic, black garlic may be more efficient at assisting your body in gaining the health advantages associated with this compound.

Roasted Garlic Vs Black Garlic

The term "roasted garlic" does not refer to the same thing as "black garlic." As was just discussed, black garlic is produced by allowing garlic cloves to sit undisturbed at a low temperature for many weeks. To make roasted garlic, just bake raw garlic at a high temperature for approximately an hour, or until it has become quite soft. The cloves of black garlic are soft and somewhat sticky, but they are still solid enough to be sliced or minced. In addition to being somewhat sour and sweet, they also have savory undertones that are not overpowering and come from the fresh garlic that is used to make them.

Cloves of roasted garlic take on a golden color and a sweet, caramelized taste. They are very soft, almost to the point of being mushy, and may be readily incorporated into mashed potatoes and salad dressings.

Varieties

There are two different types of multi-clove and solo-clove whole bulbs of black garlic. It is quite possible that you are already acquainted with the garlic that is called multi-clove. Because the skins keep each clove distinct, they need to be peeled separately.

Garlic with a solo clove, also known as single-clove garlic, is more compact in size and has a round shape. As you cut into the bulb, there is no separation from the skins once you reach the inside. It's simply a single, big, spherical clove all by itself.

Flavor

The taste of black garlic has a subtle sweetness that is reminiscent of rich molasses and a faint tang that is similar to that of tamarind or balsamic vinegar. Additionally, it has depth and umami traces of soy sauce. Its cloves are significantly sticky and have a softer texture than those of fresh garlic. During the aging process, the cloves get somewhat drier, which results in a texture that is a little chewy yet soft.

Where to get

Black garlic is readily accessible for purchase online from both major and small manufacturers, and it is also often stocked in grocery specialty shops and health food establishments.

You may get aged black garlic and fermented black garlic in a variety of forms, including entire bulbs, peeled cloves, puree, dried, and granulated forms. Find black garlic in the form of bulbs, cloves, or purees if you wish to use it in dishes in the same way that you would use conventional raw or roasted garlic. The smaller jars or bundles containing two to five bulbs of black garlic are the ones that are most often seen at retail establishments.

If you want black garlic in large quantities, it is possible to make black garlic at home by putting whole bulbs in a slow cooker or rice cooker and setting it to the low-temperature setting; however, it will take anywhere from three to six weeks for the garlic to reach its full maturity.

Where to store

Black garlic bulbs that have not been peeled may be kept at room temperature in their package as long as they have not been opened. Once the box has been opened, it should be kept in the refrigerator until the best-before or use-by date, whichever comes first. When stored properly in the refrigerator, black garlic may keep for up to one month.

Cloves of peeled black garlic, either whole or chopped, as well as purees, should be kept in the refrigerator in airtight containers or glass jars.

How to incorporate black garlic into your cooking

Black garlic, much like its fresh counterpart, may be consumed either raw or cooked. If you have full bulbs of black garlic, you will need to peel the cloves before you can use them. However, peeling black garlic cloves takes far less time than peeling fresh garlic cloves. It should not be difficult to separate the cloves from their skins. After being peeled, black garlic may be cut into pieces, minced, or mashed before being used in any dish that calls for fresh garlic.

Bear in mind, however, that black garlic does not possess the sharp taste of fresh garlic, which means that its flavor may be easily overpowered by other components. It is possible that you may need to use more black garlic than you would fresh garlic or use it in dishes with basic tastes in order to allow the black garlic's singular flavor to shine through. The following is a list of some of the uses for black garlic:

- Blend it with condiments (like mayonnaise!) as well as add flavor to potato salad or burgers.

- Include it in dishes such as salsas, spaghetti sauces, soups, and stews by stirring it in.

- Sprinkle it on pizzas and flatbreads to give them some flavor.

- It may also be used successfully in unconventional sweets, like ice cream and brownies, for example.

You might like the flavor of black garlic better than raw garlic.

6. Chapter 2.

The Mysterious History of Black Garlic

Around the year 2008, black garlic, had its moment in the spotlight. Instantaneously, it spread to all of the world's most prestigious dining establishments, and chefs competed with one another to create the black garlic dish that would top them all. But where did it come from in the first place? The history of black garlic is cloudy, and there are a few different hypotheses regarding where it could have come from. In 2009, a garlic farmer in the United Kingdom made the claim that he had created black garlic using a recipe that was 4,000 years old and originated in Korea. More contemporary accounts place the phenomenon's beginning in the early 20th century[4].

Some families in Japan and Korea assert that their ancestors have been cultivating and using black garlic for hundreds of years, which is another theory. It is likely that all of these explanations for the origin of black garlic are plausible, and that instead, black garlic was simply "rediscovered" independently numerous times throughout history. In Ayurveda, there is a widespread misconception that garlic and onion are off-limits. The origin of this misconception is unknown. Do not be afraid, and eat to your heart's content while reaping the many advantages to your health!

There are two main stories regarding the origin of black garlic, one ancient and one modern, are as dissimilar to one another as is humanly possible. You're going to hear both of these stories, and then we'll let you choose which one you think is more likely to be true.

Mark Botwright

A British farmer by the name of Mark Botwright was interested in finding out how to store the 900,000 bulbs of garlic that he cultivated so that they may be used continuously throughout the year. Suddenly, he stumbles onto an ancient Korean recipe for black garlic that dates back 4,000 years. The bulbs must be subjected to "heat and moisture for more than a month" as part of this process. He applies the process to his bulbs, and "Voila," he finds black garlic, and he is immediately enamored with the silky, sweet taste of the garlic. He then works to refine his method and keeps his discovery a well-guarded secret, going so far as to avoid divulging the original ancient source of his finding.

Scott Kim

In the year 2004, Korean inventor Scott Kim builds and patents a machine that can produce black garlic. His "machine keeps the bulbs for three weeks, during which time the controlled heat and humidity pull out natural sugars and make the cloves black." The bulbs remain on the cooling rack for one more week before being packaged. By 2008, his firm, Black Garlic Inc., had begun manufacturing the bulbs on a large scale and marketing them. At the same time that the mysterious black garlic, which had just been labeled a "super food," was making its way across the globe, many hypotheses about its beginnings were also doing the rounds. Kim remained steadfast in his assertion and said, "Contrary to what you may have been led to believe, black garlic is not an old cuisine from Korea... I am the inventor of it, and my exclusive technique is protected by three patents."

You are now familiar with the two primary hypotheses, but this is only the beginning of the fascinating complexity that lies ahead. There are further stories that are not as well known that assert it originated in Japan a few centuries ago. In yet another account, a Korean family located in Toronto has claimed that they have been fermenting black garlic in clay pots for more than a century. The family claims that they have been doing this for generations. [5] The fact that it is really tasty is not a mystery, despite the fact that no one has been successful in unearthing the truth about it (or, if they have, they are hesitant to tell it).

The cultural beginnings of black garlic

Additionally, Black Garlic has a great deal of cultural weight and importance. Many people believe that Korea was the country that was responsible for its first dissemination, even if its roots are on the Asian continent. The Koreans considered black garlic to be an effective health remedy, and they used it to cure a wide range of conditions, in addition to using it to enhance their physical power and vitality. As its reputation grew over time, black garlic began to show up in markets all over the world, including China, Vietnam, and Thailand. The ancient method for preparing black garlic consisted of placing the garlic cloves in earthenware or ceramic containers, locking the lids, and storing them in a cold, dry place for many months. This allowed the garlic to ferment on its own. There are a number of cultural beliefs associated with black garlic. In Korea, it was believed that giving the traditional six clove black garlic to women would grant the women supernatural powers and even immortality. On the other hand, in the Taoist mythology that was practiced in some communities in Vietnam and Thailand, people believed that the process of changing a Taoist's DNA required the usage of six-clove garlic. This was a notion that was maintained by certain groups. By concentrating and amplifying their vital force, this was believed to offer them immortality.

Therefore, throughout history and civilization, black garlic has been regarded as a super food since it is said to contain a number of features and advantages that are beneficial to one's health. And that assertion seems to be justified even in the present day, as a growing number of investigations and studies suggest that black garlic is, in point of fact, a Super Food[5].

Black Garlic production – The Maillard reaction or Fermentation

Fermentation is often used to describe the process by which black garlic is produced; however, there is no real fermentation that takes place during the production of black garlic.

What is fermentation?

Microorganisms such as bacteria or yeasts are responsible for the transformation of one substance into another during the fermentation process. The normally pungent enzymes found in white garlic are degraded during the aging process that produces black garlic, which takes place in an environment that is warm and humid. In contrast to the more immediate Maillard reactions, such as toasting a marshmallow, the breakdown of the garlic takes a lengthy period of time, exactly like many fermented processes. This distinguishes it from those processes.

Maillard reaction

A chemical process known as the Maillard reaction is responsible for the transformation of raw garlic into its characteristic dark color. The question now is, what exactly is the Maillard reaction? In the world of chemistry, the term "Maillard reaction" refers to the chemical reaction that takes place between amino acids and sugars in the presence of heat. This process causes food to brown and gives it a new flavor, color, and aroma. Sugar is another substance that often exists in food products, as is the case with amino acids, which are a kind of protein. During the Maillard reaction, the amino acids and sugars that are present in the food are reorganized in such a way that they reflect light in a specific manner. This is what gives the meal its characteristic brown color and texture. The Maillard reaction not only gives the food its characteristic brown color but also imparts flavor and scent to it at the same time. When frying, roasting, or otherwise preparing food in a manner that generates heat, the Maillard reaction takes place, which results in the formation of numerous molecules that give the finished product its distinctive scent. The Maillard reaction is not something that happens just in a select few foods when they are cooked; rather, it happens in almost all foods when they are cooked. Even if the flavor and scent could be different from one food item to the next, the coloring might be the same. Heat, moisture, and time are the three essential requirements for a Maillard reaction to take place. Maillard reaction takes place in the production of black garlic because it is done at a slightly high temperature, with moisture, and over a long period of time. As a result, black garlic cannot be produced apart from the Maillard process, and thus, the foods that we take pleasure in eating today would lack their distinctive flavor and scent in the absence of the Maillard reaction[6].

What is it exactly?

After doing some study on the topic, I have come to the conclusion that the Maillard reaction, which is the primary chemical reaction taking place in this scenario, is responsible for the browning of the black garlic. I am unsure as to whether or not it may also be described as having undergone the process of fermentation at the same time.

It is likely going to come down to the question of whether or not there are any microorganisms engaged in the process of breakdown. The temperatures that are required to make black garlic are reportedly high for a genuine fermentation process to take place, according to another theory that I've come across. It's possible that what we're witnessing is an enzymatic breakdown happening at the same time as the Maillard process. At the very least, the process is fairly similar to one that involves fermentation; yet, it is probably not a fermentation at all.

7. Chapter 3.

Remarkable Health Benefits Associated With Black Garlic

The health advantages of black garlic are many and may even exceed the benefits of raw garlic. In this chapter, we take a look at some of the possible health advantages that black garlic may offer. Black garlic is a harmless food product that may be used in the same manner as fresh garlic; nevertheless, the FDA has not granted approval for its usage in the medical field, and there is a general dearth of reliable clinical studies. Consult your primary care provider before beginning supplementation with black garlic. There is no evidence from clinical trials to support the use of black garlic in the treatment of any of the illnesses described in this section. The following is the data of the previous research that was conducted on animals and cell-based systems, which ought to direct any future investigative endeavors. However, the research described below should not be taken as evidence that any of the health benefits being claimed are true.

Contains more antioxidants

The fermenting procedure results in black garlic having a much higher concentration of antioxidants than raw garlic does. This is due to the fact that when black garlic ferments, the molecule known as allicin, which is responsible for the strong odor that is released when garlic is crushed, is transformed into antioxidant chemicals such as alkaloids and flavonoids. Allicin is transformed into a number of different chemicals throughout the process that transforms garlic into black garlic[7].

There are several different antioxidants in black garlic:

- **Amadori and Heyns compounds:** These are the chemicals that are generated as a result of the Maillard process. Strong antioxidants known as Amadori/Heyns compounds may be found in black garlic, which, in comparison to fresh garlic, has anywhere from 40 to 100 times more of these compounds.

- **5-hydroxymethylfurfural:** It's an anti-inflammatory compound that also functions as an antioxidant. Its name comes from its chemical structure. Because 5-HMF is produced during the fermentation process at high temperatures, black garlic contains a much greater concentration of this healthful component as compared to white garlic.

- **Organosulfur compounds:** Diallyl sulphide, diallyl disulfide, diallyl trisulfide, and diallyl tetrasulfide

- Pyruvate: It's an important chemical in black garlic that functions as both an antioxidant and an anti-inflammatory. Nitric oxide and prostaglandin E2, both of which prolong and aggravate inflammation, are both reduced as a result of this.

- **S-allylcysteine**

- **Tetrahydro-β-carbolines**

- **N-fructosyl glutamate**

- **N-fructosyl-arginine (NFA)**

- **Allixin**

- **Selenium**

- **N-alpha-(1-deoxy-d-fructose-1-yl)**

- **L-arginine**

- **Flavonoids, polyphenols, and other alkaloids**

Additionally, black garlic contains nitrogen oxide, which research has shown to have powerful anticancer and antiviral effects. In addition to that, it has an anti-inflammatory chemical known as

2-linoleoyl-glycerol. Prostaglandin E2 and cytokines, which are important in the promotion and signaling of the inflammatory response, make the process of cell death more drawn out and exacerbate it, along with swelling and other unpleasant symptoms of an allergy, infection, or other illness, are reduced to lower levels as a result.

The Mechanism of Working

Garlic is loaded with hydrogen-sulfur donating chemicals, which are essential for the development of its antioxidant effects. These compounds may be found in extremely high concentrations in garlic. Garlic has an unstable component known as allicin. This component may be transformed into organosulfur compounds, which are not only more stable but also have the ability to donate hydrogen and sulfur.

Compounds that donate hydrogen and sulfur are very necessary for antioxidant actions since doing so activates the Nfr-2 factor. When Nfr-2 factors bind to antioxidant response elements, this causes the release of a number of different enzymes:

- Heme oxygenase-1

- Superoxide dismutase

- Catalase

- Quinone-oxidoreductase-1

- Glutathione S-transferase

All of these enzymes are essential because they may turn into effective antioxidants, changing potentially harmful oxygen and nitrogen atoms into states in which they cannot combine with one another and cause major damage to cells in the human body. The antioxidant potential of black garlic may be attributed in large part to organosulfur compounds that are produced from allicin. Antioxidants are molecules that assist in protecting your cells from oxidative damage, which, if left unchecked, may lead to a variety of ailments. The majority of antioxidants that people ingest come from plant foods, including garlic. According to the findings of one research published in 2014, the level of total antioxidant activity dramatically increased in aged black garlic. According to the findings of the same research, garlic's antioxidant level peaked after 21 days of fermentation.

Regulates blood sugar

People who have diabetes and have high blood sugar are at an increased risk of serious health concerns, some of which include kidney damage, infections, and heart disease. An extract of black garlic was given to rats in a study that was conducted in 2019, and the rats were fed a diet that was high in fat and sugar. The rats that were treated with the extract of black garlic exhibited metabolic improvements such as lowered cholesterol, decreased inflammation, and regulation of appetite[8].

A previous research carried out in 2009 on diabetic rats indicated that the antioxidant properties of black garlic might help guard against the problems that are often the outcome of elevated blood sugar. In yet another experiment conducted in 2019, researchers gave rats a diet that was very heavy in fat. When compared to rats who didn't eat it, rats that did ingest black garlic had much lower levels of glucose and insulin in their blood than those that did consume it.

It is essential to keep in mind that some of these findings originated from research conducted on animals and that more research into the effectiveness of black garlic on diabetes and blood sugar levels in people is still required.

Lowers the likelihood of developing heart disease

Several studies found that black garlic helped people with slightly elevated cholesterol levels achieve healthier cholesterol levels. In a human research that lasted for 12 weeks and used placebos, 30 participants were given 6 grams of black garlic before each meal for the duration of the study. At the conclusion of the research project, the levels of HDL cholesterol, also known as "good" cholesterol, were shown to have risen when compared to the placebo group. On the other hand, there was a slight decrease in LDL, sometimes known as the "bad cholesterol".

Because of its high concentration of organosulfur compounds, black garlic also has the ability to relax blood vessels, which results in a reduction in blood pressure. Patients with high blood pressure took either two or four black garlic cloves every day over the course of the trial, which lasted for twelve weeks. It resulted in an overall reduction of 11.8 mm Hg in their blood pressure[9].

In yet another experiment involving animals, researchers discovered that giving rats a diet heavy in fat resulted in increased levels of total blood fats, triglycerides, and cholesterol. Black garlic extract helped lower these levels. The presence of these at elevated levels is often indicative of an increased risk of cardiovascular disease.

In one investigation, individuals who had coronary heart disease were given 20 grams of black garlic extract once a day for a period of six months. In comparison to those who took a placebo, individuals who ingested it had higher levels of antioxidants in their bodies and better signs of how well their hearts were functioning.

It is possible that including black garlic in your diet will help you maintain or enhance your cardiovascular health; however, further research on humans is needed to better understand the impact that black garlic supplements have on the heart.

There Is Not Enough Evidence to Support

The following alleged advantages are only substantiated by a small number of clinical research that is of poor quality. There is not enough evidence to support the use of black garlic for any of the purposes that are indicated here. Always consult a medical professional before using black garlic, and under no circumstances should you use it in lieu of anything your physician has recommended or prescribed.

Fights Inflammation

In experiments conducted on both humans and animals, black garlic was shown to reduce the effects of blood clotting brought on by platelet aggregation. An antioxidant called 5-HMF, which can be found in black garlic was used in research on human cells, and it was observed that it inhibited the activation of nuclear factor kappa B (NF-B). This molecule is responsible for regulating the production of cytokines, which help TNF- stimulated cells remain active for a longer period of time.

Cells that have been triggered by TNF- contribute to the inflammatory response, which increases blood flow, swelling, and the number of defense cells that are drawn to the location. Additionally, the number of proteins that link cells and cause blood clots was reduced. The number of cells that are responsible for inflammation and damage to cells was also reduced[10].

In a test utilizing macrophages, which are immune cells, researchers found that black garlic was able to reduce the synthesis of nitric oxide, TNF-, and prostaglandin E2, all of which are significant contributors to inflammatory responses. It was able to achieve this by lowering the levels of a number of different proteins and enzymes, in particular NO synthase, TNF-, and cyclooxygenase-2 protein.

In a study with mice, the researchers found that when the animals were given 120 mg/kg of black garlic, their blood levels of the cytokines TNF- and IL-6 were reduced. For the purpose of determining the function, if any, that black garlic plays in the reduction of inflammation in people, larger and more rigorous clinical tests will be necessary. For the time being, all that we can truly say is that including black garlic in a diet that is otherwise healthy won't do any harm.

Provides defense against allergies

Antibodies called immunoglobulin E (IgE) and mast cells are linked to the development of allergies. Both of these factors contribute to the promotion of chronic inflammation. To be more specific, a type I allergic reaction is initiated when the IgE receptor, which is found on the surface of immune cells' apical membrane is engaged.

A reduction in the levels of inflammatory enzymes (-hexosaminidase and TNF-) was seen in a cell experiment in which black garlic was administered at a concentration of 2 mg/mL. Because of this, an allergic reaction was avoided. In another cell study, the use of black garlic at a concentration of 50 g/mL inhibited key allergy-promoting molecules (prostaglandin E2, leukotriene B4, and cyclooxygenase-2) and prevented signaling (phosphorylation of Syk, phospholipase A2, and 5-lipoxygenase) that can lead to the attack of cells by immune system cells known as macrophages.

Mice that were given black garlic had a reduced allergic reaction, which was observable on their skin. Research on animals and cells suggests that black garlic may be able to reduce the markers of allergies and prevent allergic responses; however, no studies on humans have been carried out at this time[11].

Reverses Liver Damage

There is some evidence that black garlic may help protect the liver against the damage that can be caused by the liver's continuous exposure to toxins, drugs, alcohol, and infections. According to research conducted on rats, black garlic has been shown to have a preventive effect in the case of a liver injury, hence avoiding future liver damage.

Additionally, there is some evidence that black garlic might be beneficial in treating chronic illnesses. For instance, one research conducted on animals indicated that black garlic enhanced liver function in the event of persistent alcohol-induced liver damage. This was likely due to the antioxidant activity of the black garlic. In yet another experiment, rats with damaged livers were given aged black garlic, which was shown to lower levels of ALT and AST, two substances in the blood that are elevated when there is liver damage.

Due to the higher level of a chemical known as CYP2E1 in black garlic, the liver's usual activity and metabolic rate were also raised. Additionally, the black garlic was able to reduce the amount of fatty liver deposits and restore a healthy balance to the liver cell diameters[12].

Helps to Manage Weight

According to research, black garlic may considerably reduce body weight, the number of adipocyte tissues, and the amount of fat distributed in the stomach.

So how exactly can black garlic fight off those extra pounds? It is believed by scientists that it eliminates fat cells by stopping new fat cells from developing. As a result, the process by which concentrated fats are converted into fat cells is slowed down. Then, it decomposes them and turns them into energy, which means that you are less likely to gain weight after including them in your diet.

A research conducted on rats found that black garlic considerably reduced body weight, as well as stomach fat and the amount of fat cells (adipocytes). In addition, the levels of triglycerides and LDL (the "bad" cholesterol) were reduced, while the levels of HDL (the "good" cholesterol) were raised.

Enhances resistance to infection

The anti-inflammatory properties of black garlic's antioxidants make it a useful food for boosting the immune system. Antioxidants engage in the battle against free radicals and protect against oxidative stress that may cause harm to cells. If your immune system is strong, it will be able to defend your body against harmful germs and illnesses more efficiently[13].

Inhibits the growth of cancer cells

According to the findings of research, black garlic may be effective in inhibiting the growth of cancer cells. Black garlic extract was shown to have higher levels of immune-stimulating, antioxidant, and anticancer effects than raw garlic extract in a research that was conducted in test tubes using the blood of 21 participants. Within three days, the researchers observed that the black garlic extract solution was toxic to cancer cells of the lung, breast, stomach, and liver.

Researchers are looking at the possibility that some of the active chemicals in black garlic might inhibit the growth of cancer cells. This is a relatively preliminary study that has only been conducted on cells; thus, no specific conclusion can be derived from it on the influence that black garlic has on cancer in real animals or humans. A great number of chemicals show "anti-cancer" actions in cells, however, these effects cannot be seen in live systems.

Direct exposure to black garlic inhibits the production of cancer-causing signaling molecules known as JNK and p38MAPK in some cancer cells. These molecules play a significant role in the development of cancer. Cancer cells such as the A549 lung cancer cell, the HepG2 liver cancer cell, and the MCF-7 breast cancer cell are a few examples of this kind. Research is being done on black garlic and the active chemicals it contains right now in the following areas[14]:

- Leukemia

- Stomach cancer

- Colon cancer

- Endometrial cancer

According to the findings of one research, it may help inhibit the development of cancer cells in the colon. Compounds found in aged black garlic have the ability to thwart the body's production of harmful free radicals. This feature helps to restrict the proliferation of cancer cells in the body and may also assist to prevent cancer from spreading to other parts of the body. At this point in time, there is not even close to adequate data to support the use of black garlic in the prevention or treatment of cancer; nevertheless, continuous cell research is being conducted.

Stomach ulcer and cancer

Patients suffering from stomach cancer may experience cell death in the presence of high amounts of black garlic.

A cancer treatment using black garlic was discovered in one research to reduce the growth of stomach tumors in mice. In addition to this, it encourages the synthesis of two essential enzymes, both of which work to protect against oxidative damage brought on by malignant cells[15].

Reduces Memory Loss

There is some evidence that black garlic may help reduce inflammation, which, over time, can cause memory loss and a decline in brain function. The buildup of a protein molecule known as beta amyloid is thought by scientists to be the root cause of inflammation in the brain, which in turn raises the probability of developing Alzheimer's disease.

According to the findings of one research conducted on rats, black garlic has the potential to lessen brain inflammation brought on by beta amyloid and even boost short-term memory. In another one of their studies, the researchers subjected the brains of rats to oxidative stress. By administering black garlic extract to the rats, scientists were able to prevent oxidative stress from leading to memory impairment. The antioxidant known as 5-HMF, which is found in black garlic, is responsible for the deactivation of the protein chain known as nuclear factor kappa B. If this protein chain is activated above its normal levels, it might result in inflammatory disorders, autoimmune illnesses, and even malignancy. Black garlic has the ability to minimize the risk of various illnesses since it inhibits the chain that causes them.

Additionally, the protein chain is accountable for the secretion of cytokines, which are proteins that regulate immune responses and have the potential to heighten pain and initiate brain inflammation. Cytokines are also involved in conditions such as asthma, atherosclerosis, and arthritis. By inhibiting the action of the nuclear factor kappa B, black garlic is able to suppress cytokine activity.

According to the findings of a research that was carried out on macrophages, which are a kind of immune cell, black garlic may decrease inflammation by lowering the production of nitric oxide (NO) and cells that are responsible for triggering inflammation. Additionally, it inhibits the activity of proteins and enzymes that are necessary for the production of nitric oxide and inflammatory cells. This, in turn, results in fewer macrophages, which are a primary contributor to the tissue damage that is linked with persistent inflammation[16].

MSG and the Brain Cells

You are undoubtedly familiar with the spice known as MSG (monosodium glutamate). In the brain cells of rats, monosodium glutamate (MSG) caused damage to the Purkinje cells in the cerebellum and hippocampus; however, the impact of MSG on humans is unknown. Both the cerebellum and the hippocampus are essential components of the brain due to their respective roles in the regulation of muscle coordination and the maintenance of long-term memories. Extract from black garlic was able to help reduce the amount of damage produced by MSG to Purkinje cells in rats[17].

The significance of this research on rats using black garlic is unclear, particularly due to the debate around monosodium glutamate (MSG), which has been shown in several studies to have no negative effects at all. It is necessary to conduct tests on humans.

8. Chapter 4.

Production of Black Garlic

Making your own Black Garlic at home is a simple process that results in a delicious specialty ingredient. In this chapter, I'll walk you through the process of making black garlic at home using an Instant Pot, slow cooker, rice cooker, or food fermenter[4], and provide some suggestions for what you can do with the fermented garlic you make at home. The following items are required in order to make black garlic at home:

- Fresh garlic heads (whole)

- Plastic wrap

- Aluminum foil

- A rice cooker, an instant pot, a slow cooker, food fermenter, or proofer

- A place in the house that may be closed off, such as a garage or an outdoor space that is covered.

- Patience. The duration of this procedure might range from three weeks to two months since it is not a rapid one.

Establishing the garlic preparation area

A well-ventilated outside spot (that is protected from the weather), a garage, or a separate room that can be closed off from the rest of the home are all good options for positioning your Instant Pot, slow cooker, rice cooker, or food fermenter.

Why? The smell of garlic is quite pungent, particularly in the early stages of the preparation process, and it remains around for at least a week, if not longer. If you are really sensitive to strong odors, it is recommended that you set up your equipment either outdoors or in a garage that has enough ventilation.

The preparation of black garlic is rather simple; all that is required is some time and perseverance. Because it is such a time-consuming procedure, I strongly suggest that you make a large quantity. That way, you will have enough for yourself and/or give it as a gift to all of your culinary friends and family.

Making Black Garlic in an Instant Pot

1. Wrap each fresh bulb of garlic individually in a plastic wrap.

2. After that, cover the bulbs in tin foil using two separate layers.

3. Raise the garlic so that it is not touching the bottom of the Instant Pot by inserting a rack inside the appliance.

4. Place the garlic cloves that have been wrapped in foil into the Instant Pot and cover it with the lid.

5. Change the temperature setting to "warm."

6. Before beginning, make sure the timer is set to the maximum amount of time (99:59, which stands for 99 hours and 59 minutes). Because the Instant Pot will turn off after every 4 days, you will need to remember to reset it to the warm setting each time the clock runs out.

7. Take a look at the calendar and mark an upcoming date that is three weeks away. When you reach that point, you should begin inspecting the garlic heads.

How to monitor the process

- After about one month or at least three weeks, you should begin checking the progress of the garlic by using the same bulb as your "official tester."

- Remove the wrapping and take out one of the garlic cloves. Take off the thin, to evaluate the situation.

- Rewrap the bulb and place it back in the Instant Pot for an additional week if it has not yet become a darker caramel color and is still firm.

- Continue to examine the garlic once a week; it might take anywhere from three to five weeks until you have dark black garlic that is smooth and sticky to the touch.

Making Black Garlic in a Slow Cooker or Rice Cooker

The method for preparing it in a slow cooker or even a rice cooker is identical to the one for preparing it in an Instant Pot. The bulbs of garlic should be individually wrapped in plastic wrap and then in two layers of foil. Next, a rack should be placed on the floor of the container to prevent the garlic from lying directly on the bottom, and the temperature should be adjusted to "warm."

After around three weeks, you should begin testing the garlic to see whether it is ready. If it hasn't become black and soft after three weeks, rewrap it and give it another week. Garlic may be "cooked" even after it has become completely black. Because the allium loses water during fermentation, the tastes get more concentrated as the process continues.

Pros: They are popular appliances, and many of us already have them in our homes. Therefore, there is no need to purchase a new appliance, which will both cost you money and take up room in your house.

Cons: During the process, it has a tendency to consume more power, which makes it less cost-effective over time. This is particularly true if you live in a region where electricity is costly. Because your slow cooker or rice cooker will be in use for an extended period of time, you won't be able to use it for any other dishes during that time.

Before investing in anything else, it could be wise to try making black garlic in a slow cooker or rice cooker first, if you already own one of those appliances, in order to test out the technique and make black garlic on a very seldom basis.

Making Black Garlic in a food fermenter

Do you want to speed up the time it takes for fermentation by a few weeks? Try out a fermenter. This appliance has the potential to reduce in half the amount of time required to produce this black gold. These appliances come at a bit of a hefty price, but you can use them to make everything from yogurt to sweet rice using just one appliance.

As the use of black garlic becomes more widespread, an increasing number of individuals are seeking methods that are not only simple but also risk-free and economical. As a result, it shouldn't come as much of a surprise that several other kinds of black garlic "fermenters" have also found their way into store shelves.

Black garlic fermenters are small kitchen equipment that has the appearance of rice cookers, but their primary function is to facilitate the speedy and simple production of black garlic at home.

Pros: They also have a tendency to operate at relatively low costs. Black garlic fermenter is estimated to use 2.16 kW per day, which isn't a terrible amount of power when one considers that it can simultaneously produce 20-30 garlic heads.

Cons: This kitchen device isn't really intended for anything else other than turning regular garlic into black garlic since that's its only purpose. In the event that you do not regularly prepare black garlic, purchasing it and storing it might be a waste of money and unnecessary space.

Making Black Garlic in a Proofer

A proofer is a special kind of small chamber that can maintain a given temperature and level of humidity for a prolonged amount of time. Their usefulness is not limited to the process of yeast fermentation that occurs in bread dough. In addition, proofers are excellent for maintaining the proper temperatures for different types of fermentation. They are perfect for producing your own yogurt or sauerkraut in the comfort of your own home. A proofer may even be used to temper chocolate or as a slow cooker that enables cooking at an exact temperature. Both of these uses are possible because of the proofer's temperature control capabilities.

The fact that you can use your own stainless steel pans inside it makes using it as a slow cooker a fantastic option. The traditional pot that may be found in slow cookers is made of stainless steel since it is more durable than ceramic and does not have the same toxicity problems that ceramic glaze does.

The fact that a proofer requires just a little amount of power to maintain a constant temperature makes it an extremely cost-effective piece of equipment to employ.

Pros: It does an excellent job of maintaining a constant temperature. In addition to this, it can be folded up into a relatively small size, allowing it to occupy much less space while it is not in use.

Cons: The cost of the appliance itself might be considered a drawback. It's possible that you'll wind up with an expensive appliance that sits in the back of your kitchen most of the time if you don't produce bread or other fermented foods, won't use it to make yogurt or temper chocolate, etc.

What is the best way to store black garlic?

Because the process of making black garlic is actually a method of preserving food, black garlic may be stored at room temperature for two to three months, or even for a longer period of time. Black garlic should be kept in an area that is cold, dry, and dark, such as a pantry. It may be stored in glass jars or even little brown lunch bags. It is also possible to freeze or refrigerate it. It may be kept for up to three months in an unpeeled form and stored in an airtight container. To prevent the garlic from becoming dry and hard, make sure the container is absolutely sealed.

- **Refrigerator:** You can keep the garlic bulbs intact in an airtight container or jar in the refrigerator, and then remove and peel the cloves as you need them. You'll be able to keep it in this manner for up to half a year.

- **Freezer:** Freeze the garlic cloves individually or the whole garlic bulb for storage. You do not need to separate them. They may be kept in the freezer for up to a year if they are first carefully wrapped in plastic wrap and then placed in the freezer. Because it does not solidify when frozen, it may be used quite soon after being removed from the freezer.

What about the safety of the food?

Is it possible that making black garlic at home might be risky? In order to prevent the development of botulism and other poisons, the temperature has to be controlled and monitored, and the pH levels should be accurate. When it comes to the preparation of black garlic, food safety expert Dr. Brian Nummer, Ph.D., has the following to say:

"The temperature during "fermentation" MUST be at or above 135 degrees Fahrenheit (57 degrees Celsius). The risk of becoming sick from consuming spoiled food increases if this temperature control is not maintained. At temperatures slightly below 57 degrees Celsius (135 degrees Fahrenheit), bacteria that cause foodborne sickness will begin to proliferate. This includes Clostridium perfringens and Clostridium botulinum. The toxin that is generated by Clostridium botulinum is the most lethal and powerful toxin that man is aware of. Because of this, the use of a temperature data recorder is strongly suggested. The fermentation of black garlic is quite different from the fermentation of classic vegetables such as sauerkraut (cabbage) or pickles (cucumbers). At room temperature, the natural (biota) lactic acid bacteria that are present in cabbage and cucumbers quickly ferment the vegetable sugars when the vegetables are submerged in salt brine. This rapid fermentation prevents pathogens like Clostridium botulinum from expanding their populations. Once the brine reaches an acidity pH of

4.6 or lower, it is no longer possible for Clostridium botulinum to grow. The fermentation of black garlic could result in an acid fermentation, but this is not guaranteed."

If you share Brian's concerns, you should properly maintain the temperature or probably steer clear of this do-it-yourself process and instead purchase black garlic from a reputable vendor.

9. Chapter 5.

FAQs and Individual Health Concerns about Consuming Black Garlic

FAQs

Is black garlic superior to white garlic?

Which option is superior to the other depends on the things you want, and it's also much a question of personal choice. They are two quite distinct things and depending on your preferences, you could choose one over the other. I personally have a lot of appreciation for both of them and would choose one over the other depending on the particular recipe I wanted to make.

There are moments when you want the strong and pungent taste that raw garlic provides. There are instances when roasted garlic is the better option. On other occasions, the sweet and rich taste of black garlic may completely change the trajectory of a cuisine. When compared to raw white garlic, black garlic is simpler to consume on its own. This is one of the many advantages of black garlic.

If you are seeking the health advantages of garlic but have a hard time consuming enough of it, black garlic is rather pleasant to consume on its own and may help you achieve your goals. In point of fact, it contains more nutrients than raw garlic, and you could discover that you want to consume it more often due to its pleasant taste[18].

Does it have a better nutritional profile than white garlic?

Consuming black garlic instead of raw white garlic may bring additional health advantages, in addition to being more convenient to consume. Although both forms of garlic include allicin, black garlic contains much larger levels of S-Ally-Cysteine. This compound is readily absorbed by the body and is believed to be responsible for many of the health advantages associated with garlic.

According to some sources, black garlic has almost twice as many antioxidants as white garlic does. On the other hand, research indicated that the extract of black garlic had a lower anti-inflammatory potential than white garlic.

Additionally, it may help stabilize blood sugar, assist in the protection of the heart, and possibly assist in the prevention of cancer. There is some evidence that black garlic may reduce inflammation, and it may also help strengthen your immune system. Some people believe that it might even aid in the process of losing weight.

What is the recommended daily intake of black garlic?

According to some sources, the recommended dose for overall health and wellness is anything from around 2 grams per day up to a little over 10 grams per day. The weight of a clove of black garlic ranges anywhere from one to five grams on average. Therefore, aiming for one to two cloves every day is most likely a reasonable target to aspire towards.

The Individual Concerns of Consuming Black Garlic

The many forms of garlic have their own unique set of potential side effects. When consumed in food or drink, black garlic might potentially have the following concerns[19]:

- Bad breath

- A burning sensation in the mouth or in the stomach

- Flatulence, gaseousness, nausea, an unpleasant body odor, or diarrhea

- Excessive consumption may cause bleeding

- Breathing problems

The following adverse effects have been linked to the excessive topical use of black garlic:

- Damage to the skin that is comparable to a burn

- Severe skin irritation

Specific Safety Measures

- **Pregnancy and Breastfeeding:** If you are pregnant or breastfeeding, you should discuss consuming black garlic with your healthcare provider beforehand. If you are pregnant, you should not use black garlic in any topical applications since it may cause inflammation.

- **Regarding the Children:** Garlic may be safely consumed by youngsters in very low doses and for just a short period of time. It is not safe to take large dosages, and doing so may potentially be deadly. However, there have been no cases of deaths documented among youngsters who have consumed garlic in any form up to this point. It is not a good idea to put black garlic on your child's skin topically since it might cause damage that is akin to burns.

- **Bleeding:** Since garlic may raise the risk of bleeding, it should be avoided by individuals who have conditions that cause them to bleed excessively, using blood thinners, or who are recovering from surgery.

- **Diabetes:** A lower blood sugar level is possible after consuming black garlic. Garlic has been shown to lower blood sugar levels in diabetic individuals, and in some cases has even been linked to diabetic coma. If you have diabetes, you should discuss taking black garlic with your primary care physician first.

- **Stomach Upset:** Black garlic may induce gastrointestinal upset; if you have a history of stomach or digestive disorders, you should discuss consuming black garlic with your doctor.

- **Reduced Blood Pressure:** Garlic has been shown to reduce blood pressure. People who have high blood pressure may benefit from this in a positive way. Those who already have low blood pressure, on the other hand, might see a drop in blood pressure. Do not take black garlic if you have a history of low blood pressure.

Serious Adverse Reactions

The consumption of black garlic as food is not associated with any serious adverse effects and is thus regarded as safe. A very unusual instance of pneumonia has been linked to the use of black garlic, according to one study. It was not possible to tell whether or not it was an instance of poisoning or immunological response. Because there have been so few substantial human clinical studies, it is impossible to speculate about the impact that black garlic will have over the long run. There will be a significant need for further clinical tests.

10. Conclusion

Even though you are probably more used to eating raw garlic, adding black garlic to your diet may be a really tasty addition. Its gelatinous texture and somewhat sweet taste complement a few different foods well. Garlic has the functions of warming and energizing the stomach, digesting food, and cleansing, which indicates that it may aid to banish the cold that's been lingering in the stomach and help with digestion. Meals that are dark in color have the potential to strengthen the kidneys and increase their function. According to Traditional Chinese Medicine (TCM)[20], these are responsible for driving and maintaining the physiological activities of the whole body.

Black garlic may assist to ease abdominal bloating, halt diarrhea, reduce swelling, and expel toxins to treat skin boils and ulcers. It can also aid to stimulate the spleen's function. In addition, it eliminates the parasitic worms that cause skin illnesses. In fact black garlic is a nutrient dense super food, give it a try!

11. References

1.	Tahir, Z., et al., *Comparative study of nutritional properties and antioxidant activity of raw and fermented (black) garlic.* International Journal of Food Properties, 2022. **25**(1): p. 116-127.

2.	Ryu, J.H. and D. Kang, *Physicochemical properties, biological activity, health benefits, and general limitations of aged black garlic: A review.* Molecules, 2017. **22**(6): p. 919.

3.	Lee, Y.-M., et al., *Antioxidant effect of garlic and aged black garlic in animal model of type 2 diabetes mellitus.* Nutrition research and practice, 2009. **3**(2): p. 156-161.

4.	Kimura, S., et al., *Black garlic: A critical review of its production, bioactivity, and application.* Journal of Food and Drug Analysis, 2017. **25**(1): p. 62-70.

5.	Toledano-Medina, M.A., et al., *Evolution of some physicochemical and antioxidant properties of black garlic whole bulbs and peeled cloves.* Food Chemistry, 2016. **199**: p. 135-139.

6.   Hodge, J.E., *Dehydrated Foods, Chemistry of Browning Reactions in Model Systems.* Journal of Agricultural and Food Chemistry, 1953. **1**(15): p. 928-943.

7.   Lee, Y.-M., et al., *Antioxidant effect of garlic and aged black garlic in animal model of type 2 diabetes mellitus.* Nutr Res Pract, 2009. **3**(2): p. 156-161.

8.   Jung, E.-S., et al., *Reduction of blood lipid parameters by a 12-wk supplementation of aged black garlic: A randomized controlled trial.* Nutrition, 2014. **30**(9): p. 1034-1039.

9.   Jeong, Y.Y., et al., *Comparison of Anti-Oxidant and Anti-Inflammatory Effects between Fresh and Aged Black Garlic Extracts.* Molecules, 2016. **21**(4): p. 430.

10.   Ha, A.W., T. Ying, and W.K. Kim, *The effects of black garlic (Allium satvium) extracts on lipid metabolism in rats fed a high fat diet.* Nutr Res Pract, 2015. **9**(1): p. 30-36.

11.   Itoh, T., et al., *Inhibitory effect of xanthones isolated from the pericarp of Garcinia mangostana L. on rat basophilic leukemia RBL-2H3 cell degranulation.* Bioorganic & Medicinal Chemistry, 2008. **16**(8): p. 4500-4508.

12.   *Hepatoprotective Effect of Aged Black Garlic on Chronic Alcohol-Induced Liver Injury in Rats.* Journal of Medicinal Food, 2011. **14**(7-8): p. 732-738.

13.   Imai, J., et al., *Antioxidant and Radical Scavenging Effects of Aged Garlic Extract and its Constituents.* Planta Med, 1994. **60**(05): p. 417-420.

14.   Purev, U., M.J. Chung, and D.-H. Oh, *Individual differences on immunostimulatory activity of raw and black garlic extract in human primary immune cells.* Immunopharmacology and Immunotoxicology, 2012. **34**(4): p. 651-660.

15.   Dong, M., et al., *Aged black garlic extract inhibits Ht29 colon cancer cell growth via the PI3K/Akt signaling pathway.* Biomed Rep, 2014. **2**(2): p. 250-254.

16.   Farombi, E.O. and O.O. Onyema, *Monosodium glutamate-induced oxidative damage and genotoxicity in the rat: modulatory role of vitamin C, vitamin E and quercetin.* Human & Experimental Toxicology, 2006. **25**(5): p. 251-259.

17.   Hermawati, E., D.C.R. Sari, and G. Partadiredja, *The effects of black garlic ethanol extract on the spatial memory and estimated total number of pyramidal cells of the hippocampus of monosodium glutamate-exposed adolescent male Wistar rats.* Anatomical Science International, 2015. **90**(4): p. 275-286.

18.   Ahmed, T. and C.-K. Wang, *Black Garlic and Its Bioactive Compounds on Human Health Diseases: A Review.* Molecules, 2021. **26**(16): p. 5028.

19.   Ma, L., et al., *Effects of Anaerobic Fermentation on Black Garlic Extract by Lactobacillus: Changes in Flavor and Functional Components.* Frontiers in

Nutrition, 2021. **8**.

20.   Kim, J., et al., *A comparative study on the antioxidative and anti-allergic activities of fresh and aged black garlic extracts.* International Journal of Food Science & Technology, 2012. **47**.

www.ingramcontent.com/pod-product-compliance
Lightning Source LLC
Chambersburg PA
CBHW051703250726

48653CB00007B/2828